Arthritis Diet

A Beginner's Step-by-Step Guide with Top Recipes: Anti-Inflammatory Diet

mf

copyright © 2019 Bruce Ackerberg

All rights reserved No part of this book may be reproduced, or stored in a retrieval system, or transmitted in any form or by any means, electronic, mechanical, photocopying, recording, or otherwise, without express written permission of the publisher.

Disclaimer

By reading this disclaimer, you are accepting the terms of the disclaimer in full. If you disagree with this disclaimer, please do not read the guide.

All of the content within this guide is provided for informational and educational purposes only, and should not be accepted as independent medical or other professional advice. The author is not a doctor, physician, nurse, mental health provider, or registered nutritionist/dietician. Therefore, using and reading this guide does not establish any form of a physician-patient relationship.

Always consult with a physician or another qualified health provider with any issues or questions you might have regarding any sort of medical condition. Do not ever disregard any qualified professional medical advice or delay seeking that advice because of anything you have read in this guide. The information in this guide is not intended to be any sort of medical advice and should not be used in lieu of any medical advice by a licensed and qualified medical professional.

The information in this guide has been compiled from a variety of known sources. However, the author cannot attest to or guarantee the accuracy of each source and thus should not be held liable for any errors or omissions.

You acknowledge that the publisher of this guide will not be held liable for any loss or damage of any kind incurred as a result of this guide or the reliance on any information provided within this guide. You acknowledge and agree that you assume all risk and responsibility for any action you undertake in response to the information in this guide.

Using this guide does not guarantee any particular result (e.g., weight loss or a cure). By reading this guide, you acknowledge that there are no guarantees to any specific outcome or results you can expect.

All product names, diet plans, or names used in this guide are for identification purposes only and are the property of their respective owners. The use of these names does not imply endorsement. All other trademarks cited herein are the property of their respective owners.

Where applicable, this guide is not intended to be a substitute for the original work of this diet plan and is, at most, a supplement to the original work for this diet plan and never a direct substitute. This guide is a personal expression of the facts of that diet plan.

Where applicable, persons shown in the cover images are stock photography models and the publisher has obtained the rights to use the images through license agreements with third-party stock image companies.

Table of Contents

Introduction	7
What Is Arthritis?	9
Causes of Arthritis	9
Symptoms of Arthritis	11
Medical Treatments	13
Lifestyle Changes to Manage Arthritis	14
The Arthritis Diet	17
Principles of Arthritis Diet	17
Benefits of Arthritis Diet	19
Disadvantages of the Arthritis Diet	21
A Step-by-Step Guide to Prevent Arthritis	23
Step 1: Seek Professional Diagnosis and Interventions	23
Step 2: Eat the Right Food	24
Food that should be avoided	31
Step 3: Weight Management	33
Step 4: Sweat It Out!	36
Endurance exercises or Aerobics	37
Strengthening exercises	37
Range-of-motion exercises	38
Body awareness exercises	38
Daily activities	38
Common mistakes to avoid during exercises:	39
Step 5: Seek Complementary Therapies & Home Remedies	42
7-Day Sample Meal Plan	46
Simple Recipes for People with Arthritis	49
Lemon Rosemary Chicken	50
Mediterranean Vegetables	52
Poached Eggs with Curry Potatoes	54
Gingerbread Oatmeal	56

Turmeric Ginger Oatmeal	58
Kale and Avocado Smoothie	60
Quinoa and Black Bean Salad	62
Salmon with Walnut-Parsley Pesto	64
Sweet Potato and Chickpea Curry	66
Salmon with Walnut-Parsley Pesto, Spinach, Apple, and Walnut Salad	68
Broccoli and Almond Soup	71
Conclusion	**74**
FAQ	**77**
References and Helpful Links	**80**

Introduction

The main purpose of this guide is to help you beat arthritis and its symptoms. Arthritis is a disease which is characterized by mild to severe pain, stiffness, tenderness, soreness, redness, and muscle weakness around joints. Joint pain is also known as arthralgia. A single joint disorder is called monoarthritis. When 2-3 joints are affected, it is called oligoarthritis. When it involves four or more joints, it becomes polyarthritis.

Arthritis is the leading cause of disability for many people around the world. It affects young and old, male and female, and the aging or elderly. There are about a hundred types of arthritis. They all affect the ability of the person to move and use other functions of joints.

The most common types of arthritis are osteoarthritis (affects the hands, hips, knees, and spine), rheumatoid arthritis (an autoimmune disease that affects joint linings), gout (condition caused by deposition of uric acid crystals in joints), fibromyalgia (pain in musculoskeletal system), lupus (a chronic inflammatory condition where the immune system attacks its tissues) and spondylitis (a condition that occurs in the spine and affects other joints).

There is no exact cure for arthritis. However, there are treatments and anti-inflammatory diet plans that can slow down its debilitating effects. This guide will give you essential tips on how to combat the agonizing pains of arthritis.

In this guide, we will talk about the following;

- What is Arthritis?
- Symptoms, Causes, and Lifestyle Changes to Manage Arthritis
- A step-by-step guide to Prevent Arthritis
- The Arthritis Diet
- 7- Day Sample Meal Plan
- Sample Recipes

This guide is a step-by-step guide for beginners who are looking for effective ways to treat or prevent arthritis. Every chapter provides a vital step towards freedom from joint pain. The last chapter gives you simple, healthy, and easy-to-prepare recipes. Keep reading to learn more about the different types of arthritis, their symptoms, causes, and management techniques.

What Is Arthritis?

Arthritis is a common condition that affects millions of people worldwide. It is characterized by inflammation of the joints, which can lead to pain, stiffness, and decreased mobility. However, arthritis is not a single disease but rather an umbrella term used to describe over 100 different types of joint disorders.

Some forms of arthritis are caused by wear and tear on the joints over time, while others are the result of an autoimmune response or other underlying health conditions. The most common types of arthritis include osteoarthritis, rheumatoid arthritis, gout, fibromyalgia, lupus, and spondylitis.

Causes of Arthritis

Arthritis, a complex condition involving inflammation of the joints, has several causes that can vary depending on the specific type of arthritis. Broadly, these causes can be categorized into a few key areas:

- *Genetic Factors*: Many types of arthritis, such as rheumatoid arthritis, have a genetic component, meaning they can run in families. Certain genes can make individuals more susceptible to environmental factors that may trigger arthritis.

- ***Immune System Dysfunction***: In autoimmune forms of arthritis, such as rheumatoid arthritis and psoriatic arthritis, the body's immune system mistakenly attacks its tissues, particularly the synovium, which is the lining of the membranes surrounding the joints. This immune response causes inflammation and can result in joint damage.
- ***Wear and Tear***: Osteoarthritis, the most common form of arthritis, results from wear and tear on the joints over time. This can be due to aging, but also from obesity, which puts extra stress on the joints, particularly those that bear weight, such as the hips and knees.
- ***Infections***: Certain infections can lead to arthritis by directly infecting the joints or triggering an immune response that affects the joints. Reactive arthritis is an example, where arthritis develops after an infection in another part of the body, such as the intestines, genitals, or urinary tract.
- ***Metabolic Issues***: Gout, another type of arthritis, occurs when there is an accumulation of urine crystals in the joint, causing inflammation and intense pain. This can happen if the body produces too much uric acid or if it has difficulty getting rid of it.

- ***Injuries***: Previous joint injuries can increase the risk of developing arthritis in that particular joint. The damage from the injury can lead to degenerative changes in the joint, leading to arthritis over time.

Understanding the underlying causes of arthritis is crucial for diagnosis and guiding treatment options. While some factors like genetics cannot be changed, others, such as lifestyle choices that affect the immune system, weight, and joint health, can be managed to reduce the risk or severity of arthritis.

Symptoms of Arthritis

The symptoms of arthritis can vary depending on the type and severity of the condition, but there are several common signs that individuals may experience. These include:

- ***Joint Pain***: One of the most frequent symptoms, joint pain can range from mild to severe and can be a constant or intermittent issue. The pain is often a result of inflammation within the joint or the wearing away of the cartilage that cushions the ends of the bones.
- ***Stiffness***: Many people with arthritis notice stiffness in their joints, particularly after periods of inactivity or upon waking in the morning. This stiffness can limit the range of motion, making it difficult to perform certain movements or tasks.

- ***Swelling***: Inflammation can cause the affected joints to swell, feel warm, and appear red. Swelling can further restrict movement and contribute to discomfort.
- ***Reduced Range of Motion***: Arthritis can lead to a decreased ability to move the affected joints through their full range of motion. This can affect daily activities and diminish an individual's quality of life.
- ***General Feeling of Unwell***: Besides the direct symptoms affecting the joints, individuals with arthritis may also experience a general feeling of being unwell, which can include fatigue and a decreased appetite.
- ***Other Symptoms***: Depending on the specific type of arthritis, other symptoms may also be present. For example, rheumatoid arthritis can cause scaly, itchy skin, changes to fingers and toenails, rashes, fever, weight loss, and hair loss in spots or around the hairline. Osteoarthritis, on the other hand, primarily affects the joints' function and comfort.

It's important for individuals experiencing these symptoms to consult a healthcare professional for an accurate diagnosis and appropriate treatment plan. Early intervention can help manage symptoms, reduce damage to the joints, and maintain quality of life.

Medical Treatments

Medical treatments for arthritis aim to reduce symptoms and improve quality of life. These treatments include:

1. **Medications**:
    - *Pain Relievers*: Over-the-counter (OTC) pain relievers such as acetaminophen, aspirin, ibuprofen, and naproxen can help relieve pain. Prescription pain medications may be recommended for more severe pain.
    - *Nonsteroidal Anti-Inflammatory Drugs (NSAIDs)*: These drugs, available OTC or by prescription, help reduce both pain and inflammation. Examples include ibuprofen, naproxen, and celecoxib.
    - *Corticosteroids*: Medications like prednisone can be taken orally or injected directly into a joint to quickly reduce inflammation and pain.
    - *Disease-Modifying Antirheumatic Drugs (DMARDs)*: These are often prescribed for rheumatoid arthritis and other autoimmune forms of arthritis to slow the progression of the disease. Examples include methotrexate, leflunomide, hydroxychloroquine, and sulfasalazine.
    - *Biologic Response Modifiers*: A subset of DMARDs, these drugs target specific steps in

the inflammatory process. They are usually prescribed for patients who have not responded well to traditional DMARDs.
2. **Physical Therapy**: Tailored exercises can help improve the range of motion and strengthen the muscles surrounding joints, which can alleviate symptoms and reduce the burden on joints.
3. **Lifestyle Modifications**: Changes such as weight loss, a healthy diet, and regular exercise can significantly impact symptom management and overall health.
4. **Surgical Treatments**: In cases where medical treatments do not sufficiently relieve symptoms, surgical options like joint repair, joint replacement, or joint fusion may be considered.
5. **Alternative Therapies**: Some people find relief from symptoms with acupuncture, massage, or dietary supplements. However, it's important to discuss these options with a healthcare provider to ensure they won't interfere with other treatments.

These treatments can be used alone or in combination, depending on the type of arthritis, its severity, and the individual's overall health and preferences.

Lifestyle Changes to Manage Arthritis

Managing arthritis effectively often involves making several lifestyle changes that can help reduce symptoms, improve joint function, and enhance overall quality of life. Here are some key lifestyle adjustments recommended for individuals with arthritis:

1. ***Regular Exercise***: Engaging in regular physical activity helps strengthen the muscles around your joints, maintain bone strength, and increase flexibility. Low-impact exercises such as walking, swimming, or cycling are particularly beneficial.
2. ***Healthy Diet***: Consuming a balanced diet rich in fruits, vegetables, whole grains, and lean proteins can help manage inflammation and maintain a healthy weight. Foods high in antioxidants and those rich in omega-3 fatty acids, such as fish, nuts, and seeds, are especially recommended. Incorporating vegetables that are high in vitamin K, such as broccoli, spinach, lettuce, kale, and cabbage, may also lower markers of inflammation in the bloodstream.
3. ***Weight Management***: Maintaining a healthy weight reduces the stress on weight-bearing joints, which can alleviate pain and prevent further joint damage. Even modest weight loss can significantly impact symptom relief.
4. ***Adequate Rest***: Ensuring you get enough rest is crucial, as it allows your body to recover and repair itself. Balance activity with periods of rest, and ensure you get quality sleep each night.

5. ***Limiting Alcohol and Quitting Smoking***: Reducing alcohol intake and quitting smoking can have positive effects on your arthritis management. Smoking can aggravate inflammatory conditions, while excessive alcohol consumption can interfere with medications and exacerbate symptoms.
6. ***Stress Management***: Chronic stress can worsen arthritis symptoms, so incorporating stress-reduction techniques such as deep breathing, meditation, yoga, or tai chi can be beneficial.
7. ***Physical Therapy***: Working with a physical therapist can provide tailored exercises to improve range of motion, strengthen muscles, and reduce pain without overburdening the joints.
8. ***Protecting Your Joints***: Use adaptive tools and devices designed to help protect your joints during daily activities. Learning proper body mechanics and ways to distribute pressure can also help.

By incorporating these lifestyle changes, individuals with arthritis can often see a significant improvement in their symptoms and overall quality of life.

The Arthritis Diet

Arthritis diet is a crucial component of managing arthritis symptoms and improving overall health. A healthy diet can help individuals with arthritis maintain a healthy weight, reduce inflammation, and provide essential nutrients for joint health.

Principles of Arthritis Diet

The arthritis diet, often associated with anti-inflammatory properties and principles similar to the Mediterranean diet, focuses on foods that can help reduce inflammation and improve overall health. Here are the key principles of the arthritis diet:

1. ***Eat Plenty of Fruits and Vegetables***: These are high in antioxidants, vitamins, and minerals, which can help reduce inflammation. Aim for a variety of colors to get a wide range of nutrients.
2. ***Incorporate Whole Grains***: Whole grains like oats, brown rice, and whole wheat bread are rich in fiber, which can help lower levels of an inflammatory marker called C-reactive protein.

3. ***Choose Lean Protein Sources***: Incorporate lean meats, fish, and plant-based proteins such as beans and lentils. Fish, especially those high in omega-3 fatty acids like salmon, mackerel, and sardines, are particularly beneficial for reducing inflammation.
4. ***Include Healthy Fats***: The diet emphasizes the importance of healthy fats, particularly those found in olive oil, avocados, nuts, and seeds. Olive oil, a staple of the Mediterranean diet, contains oleocanthal, which has properties similar to nonsteroidal anti-inflammatory drugs.
5. ***Limit Processed Foods and Sugars***: Processed foods and added sugars can increase inflammation in the body. Reducing their intake is crucial for managing arthritis symptoms.
6. ***Stay Hydrated***: Drinking plenty of water is essential for overall health and can help keep joints lubricated.
7. ***Moderate Alcohol Consumption***: If alcohol is consumed, it should be in moderation. Some studies suggest that red wine may have anti-inflammatory effects due to its resveratrol content.
8. ***Spices and Herbs***: Incorporating anti-inflammatory spices and herbs like turmeric, ginger, and garlic can add flavor to meals while potentially reducing inflammation.

Adopting these dietary principles can help manage arthritis symptoms by reducing inflammation, improving joint health, and enhancing overall well-being.

Benefits of Arthritis Diet

The arthritis diet, focused on reducing inflammation and improving joint health through nutrition, offers several benefits for individuals dealing with various forms of arthritis.

Here are some of the key benefits:

1. ***Reduction in Inflammation***: The diet emphasizes foods known to reduce inflammation, such as fruits, vegetables, whole grains, and omega-3 fatty acids. Lowering inflammation can help reduce joint pain and stiffness.
2. ***Improved Joint Health***: Nutrients found in the recommended foods, like vitamin K in green leafy vegetables and omega-3 fatty acids in fatty fish, are essential for maintaining healthy joints and can contribute to improved mobility and reduced pain.
3. ***Weight Management***: By focusing on whole foods and limiting processed items and sugars, the arthritis diet can help individuals achieve or maintain a healthy weight. Being overweight puts extra stress on joints, particularly those that bear weight, so weight management is crucial for reducing symptoms.

4. ***Enhanced Overall Health***: This diet plan is rich in antioxidants, vitamins, minerals, and fiber, which support a healthy immune system and can improve overall health. It aligns closely with heart-healthy diets, potentially reducing the risk of cardiovascular diseases.
5. ***Increased Energy Levels***: Foods included in the arthritis diet can provide more steady energy levels throughout the day, avoiding the spikes and crashes often associated with high-sugar and processed foods.
6. ***Better Digestive Health***: High fiber content from whole grains, fruits, and vegetables supports good digestive health, which can also impact inflammation and immune function positively.
7. ***Reduced Risk of Chronic Diseases***: The principles of the arthritis diet overlap significantly with those recommended for preventing and managing other chronic diseases, such as diabetes, heart disease, and certain cancers.

By adhering to the principles of the arthritis diet, individuals can not only manage their arthritis symptoms more effectively but also enjoy a range of health benefits that contribute to a higher quality of life.

Disadvantages of the Arthritis Diet

While the arthritis diet, focused on reducing inflammation and supporting joint health through nutrition, offers numerous benefits, it's important to acknowledge that there may be some disadvantages or challenges associated with it. However, it's crucial to note that for most individuals, the advantages significantly outweigh these potential drawbacks.

- **Restrictive Elements**: For some people, the diet may feel restrictive, especially if it involves cutting out foods they enjoy, such as certain dairy products, processed foods, or sweets. This can make adherence challenging over the long term.
- **Initial Adjustment Period**: Transitioning to an arthritis-friendly diet may require an adjustment period, particularly for those used to a diet high in processed foods and sugars. Initial cravings and a sense of deprivation may occur.
- **Cost Considerations**: Opting for whole, unprocessed foods, organic produce, and high-quality sources of protein might increase grocery bills. While this isn't universally true, perceived higher costs can be a barrier for some individuals.
- **Time and Effort**: Preparing fresh meals daily requires more time and effort than opting for pre-packaged or processed options. Busy lifestyles may make this challenging for some people.

- ***Social and Cultural Adjustments***: Dietary changes might affect social interactions, particularly during dining out or attending events where food choices are limited. It may also require adjustments within households where not everyone is following the same dietary guidelines.

While there are certain challenges associated with adopting the arthritis diet, the benefits in terms of symptom management, overall health improvement, and enhanced quality of life make it a worthwhile endeavor for many individuals dealing with arthritis.

A Step-by-Step Guide to Prevent Arthritis

Now that we have discussed the basics of the arthritis diet, let's look at how you can start incorporating these changes into your daily life. Here is a step-by-step guide to help you get started on preventing and managing arthritis:

Step 1: Seek Professional Diagnosis and Interventions

The initial and vital step towards arthritis management is to seek a diagnosis from a rheumatologist, a doctor with special training in arthritis treatment, and other related diseases.

A meeting between you and a doctor is very important. At this stage, your doctor will evaluate your condition, examine your joints, ask questions, and assess the symptoms' history. He may even recommend laboratory tests (urine, joint fluid, and blood) and subject you to an X-ray before making a diagnosis. An early and accurate diagnosis prevents disability or irreversible damage in the joints caused by arthritis.

Sometimes, you need more than just a rheumatologist to manage arthritis. A team of health care professionals which includes an orthopedic surgeon, physiotherapist, orthotist, occupational therapist, dietitian, chiropractor, psychologist, and nurse specialist can help you beat the disease by creating a cure plan.

A cure plan involves medications, exercise, proper rest and sleep, physical therapy, a healthy diet, and possible surgery options. A surgical procedure becomes necessary if the disease has damaged the nerves of the spine. A regular check-up and monitoring of your joint condition are important to assess the effectiveness of the treatment or medication. A joint disease that is not treated properly brings health complications and non-joint manifestations of other diseases.

If you are experiencing discomfort or pain in the joints, don't ignore it. Visit your doctor or seek the help of a rheumatologist and get a diagnosis to evaluate the stage of your joint pains.

Do not allow arthritis to keep you from living a healthy and active lifestyle.

Step 2: Eat the Right Food

Is there an effective arthritic or anti-inflammatory diet?

Many studies showed that certain foods and ingredients have anti-inflammatory properties, thereby helping prevent symptoms that can cause arthritis. This chapter is about eating the right type of food and avoiding those that trigger inflammation, and elevate the level of uric acid.

According to health experts, what you eat can influence the progression or alleviation of arthritic symptoms. The food you eat plays a major role in arthritis management.

Here is a simple guide:

Fish

The Academy of Nutrition and Dietetics and the American Heart Association recommend eating 3-4 ounces of fish at least 2 times a week. More is always better. Fish contains high amounts of omega-3s. This fatty acid lowers the level of active inflammatory proteins- the interleukin 6 and the C-reactive protein (CRP).

The best sources are salmon, scallops, tuna, anchovies, herring, sardines, and other cold-water fish.

You can also take fish oil supplements. A 600-1000 mg. of fish oil every day aids in relieving pain, joint stiffness, swelling, and tenderness.

Fruits and Vegetables

Fruits and vegetables are packed with antioxidants. These powerful chemicals neutralize free radicals. Antioxidants also act as natural defense agents of the body.

Remember that darker fruits contain more antioxidants.

- Cherries contain anthocyanins.
- Citrus fruits like limes, oranges, and grapefruits are packed with vitamin C. This vitamin prevents inflammation and keeps joints healthy.
- Purple and red fruits like raspberries, strawberries, blackberries, and blueberries provide anti-inflammatory benefits.

Consuming vegetables high in Vitamin K can significantly reduce the levels of inflammatory markers in the blood. Examples are kale, broccoli, cabbage, lettuce, and spinach.

Nine or more servings of fruits and veggies a day are highly recommended. One serving is equivalent to 2 cups of raw green, leafy veggies or 1 cup of fruit (or other types of vegetables).

Nuts and Seeds

Many studies confirm the important role of nuts in an anti-inflammatory diet. In 2oo1, a Circulation journal article attested to the fact that vitamin B6 in nuts lowers the level of inflammatory markers in the body.

Another study published in The American Journal of Clinical Nutrition showed that people who regularly have nuts in their diet have a 51% lower risk level to suffering and dying from inflammatory diseases including rheumatoid arthritis.

Nuts are rich in monounsaturated fat, a potent inflammation-fighting type of fat that also promotes weight loss. They contain a great amount of protein and fiber.

The best sources are almonds, walnuts, pistachios, and pine nuts.

The daily recommended serving is 1.5 ounces. One ounce equates to a handful. However, do not forget that more is not always better. Limit your consumption within the recommended amount.

Whole Grains

Whole grains contain fibers that can lower the level of C-reactive protein, an inflammatory marker in the blood.

The best sources are oatmeal, brown rice, whole-wheat flour, quinoa, bulgur, and other grain kernel varieties.

The recommended daily serving is 6 ounces with at least 3 ounces coming from whole grains. One ounce of whole grain is equivalent to 1 slice of whole-wheat bread or ½ cup of cooked brown rice.

Beans

Beans contain phytonutrients and fiber that help in the reduction of CRP levels. High CRP level indicates active inflammation and infection that cause rheumatoid arthritis.

The best sources are red kidney beans, pinto beans, and small red beans. They are excellent sources of protein that promote muscle health.

The recommended serving is one cup, 2 times a week. One cup contains 15 grams of beans. More can be beneficial.

Olive Oil

Olive oil contains oleocanthal, a heart-healthy fat that produces similar effects to non-steroidal, anti-inflammatory drugs. It reduces the potential risk of damage to joint cartilage. Oleocanthal also inhibits the production of COX enzymes- COX-1 and COX-2. These enzymes can greatly reduce pain sensitivity and hinder inflammatory processes in the body.

The best source is extra virgin olive oil which contains natural nutrients.

Recommended consumption is 2-3 tablespoons every day.

Tea

Green, white, black, and oolong tea are loaded with polyphenol compounds that protect the body against arthritis and boost the health of the immune system. Tea revs up the ability of T-cells to react against viral and bacterial infections.

Green tea is believed to be more beneficial compared to other types of tea drinks. In 2015, the International Journal of Rheumatic Diseases published an article about the superiority of anti-inflammatory properties of green tea compared to black tea.

Green tea contains potent antioxidants that block the production of joint-damaging molecules in the body. It has an EGCF substance that blocks interleukin-1, an inflammatory cell that can damage cartilage. By blocking the compound, the progression of arthritis is greatly reduced. It can effectively change various immune responses that reduce the level of arthritic pains.

To sustain the level of polyphenols in the blood, drinking 7-8 cups of tea every day is recommended. The best way to maximize the potency of polyphenol is to steep a bag of tea for 5 minutes in boiled water.

Foods from the Allium Family

Onions, garlic, and leeks are beneficial foods from the allium family. They contain diallyl disulfide, which limits the production of enzymes that can damage the cartilage.

Include these foods in your daily meal preparation or eat raw if you can.

Vitamin E-packed foods

Vitamin E is an antioxidant that reduces inflammation.

The best natural sources are avocado, peanut, spinach, sunflower seeds, almonds, and wheat germ oil.

- One piece of avocado provides 20% of the required daily need of Vitamin E.
- One cup of almonds gives twice the amount of vitamin E you need for the day.
- One-fourth cup of peanuts gives 20% of vitamin E.
- One-half cup of spinach provides 16% of the Vitamin E requirement.
- One tablespoon of wheat germ oil provides 100% of your daily Vitamin E consumption.

Grass-fed beef, Fermented dairy products, and Organic poultry

They all contain omega-3 fatty acids and medium-chain saturated fats which enhance the functions of the immune system, produce good hormones, and sustain the health of cell membranes.

Recommended consumption is eating small amounts every day to maximize extraction of key nutrients as well as avoid digestion troubles.

Curcumin

Curcumin is the active ingredient of turmeric. It contains large amounts of anti-inflammatory compounds that can effectively treat all types of arthritis.

500 mg. A daily dose is recommended to fight inflammation.

Food that should be avoided

Cutting back on the consumption of the following food reduces inflammation and restores the natural defense ability of the body. Total elimination will bring more health benefits.

Processed food

Avoid prepared frozen meals snacks, and baked goods because they use trans-fats to facilitate the process of preservation. This type of fat can cause systemic inflammation.

Red Meat

Red meat is rich in saturated fats that can trigger inflammation and high cholesterol conditions. It also contains an advanced glycation end-product (AGE's) substance which destroys certain proteins in the body.

AGE is a type of toxin that is produced when foods are cooked at a very high temperature (grilled, fried, roasted, pasteurized, or broiled).

Fried Foods

Fried chicken, French fries, donuts, fried meat, and other fried food contain trans-fats and AGEs (advanced glycation end-products) that trigger inflammation.

High-Carbs foods

Refined grains such as white pasta, crackers, and white bread spike the level of blood glucose and inflammation markers.

Refined Sugar

Foods that use high amounts of refined sugar are chocolates, pastries, soda, fruit juices, and candies. Sugar forms include fructose, maltose, sucrose, or corn syrup.

Sugar triggers the production of cytokines and AGE which in turn causes body inflammation.

Dairy Products

Cheese, cream cheese, margarine, butter, and mayonnaise contain AGEs and saturated fats, the two triggers of body inflammation.

Some dairy products have certain types of protein that irritate joints.

Alcohol

Too much alcohol in the body can cause gout. Cut back on alcohol consumption to prevent joint pains.

Salt and Preservatives

Foods that contain high amounts of sodium and preservatives cause joint inflammation.

Always read product labels to avoid buying foods with excessive additives and preservatives.

Step 3: Weight Management

Obese and overweight people have a greater risk of getting arthritis. This is due to the obvious fact that extra weight strains joints in the ankles, spine, hips, knees, and feet. Another reason is the increased production of inflammatory mediators in fat tissues that bring joint problems.

If you are already having joint pains from being overweight, it's time to lose excess fats to slow down the progression of arthritis. Losing weight is necessary to beat arthritis.

Benefits of losing weight:

1. **Decreased joint pressure**

    Weight loss improves joint functions, especially on the knees. Knee joints are the most mechanically pressured joints. Losing one pound removes four pounds of knee pressure.

2. **Reduced pain and inflammation**

   A lighter body suffers lesser pain. Weight loss effectively lowers inflammation levels and improves joint condition. A combination of a healthy diet and exercise helps the body eliminate fats.

   Fats trigger the production and release of pro-inflammatory compounds in the body, one of them is IL-6 or interleukin-6. Without a great amount of fats to trigger the release of these chemicals, inflammation and pain are greatly reduced.

3. **Improved Health**

   Weight loss significantly improves the well-being and quality of life of an individual. Without chronic pains, life becomes better.

4. **Lower risk of chronic diseases**

   Weight loss lowers the potential risk of diabetes and cancer. A moderate weight loss of 14 pounds leads to a 58% decrease in the risk of type-2 diabetes.

   It also decreases the risk of developing chronic rheumatoid arthritis and osteoarthritis.

5. **Reduces heart disease and stroke dangers**

   Weight loss lowers blood pressure and cholesterol levels. A 5-10 pound weight loss reduces the risk of stroke and heart disease. A study published in the Annals of Rheumatic Disease in 2013 showed that painful hand osteoarthritis is closely associated with heart disease.

6. Prevents Sleep Apnea and other Sleep disorders

The musculoskeletal pains affect and interfere with a good night's sleep which causes chronic insomnia. Weight management programs significantly improve sleep patterns.

A ten percent decrease in total body weight has long-term effects on sleep apnea. It makes breathing better and easier.

7. Cost-saving

Arthritis and other joint problems are costly diseases. Medication and treatment programs are expensive. According to the Centers for Disease Control and Prevention (CDC), about $128 billion annually is spent to cure arthritis. The increasing cost of medication affects aging people who are more prone to joint pain.

To gain all these benefits, start losing weight.

Step 4: Sweat It Out!

Do not allow arthritis to immobilize you. Keep going and moving by sweating out daily. Even moderate types of exercise can ease joint pains and maintain flexibility.

Physical exercise is an important part of weight management programs to treat arthritis. However, it is necessary to follow the recommendation of your healthcare team or attending doctor on the type of exercise that suits your condition.

People with arthritis who regularly exercise show better muscle strength and higher levels of fitness. Their moods improved and they were able to perform their daily tasks again without pain.

Benefits of exercise:

- Strengthens muscles around joints
- Provides more energy to combat fatigue
- Improves balance
- Maintains bone strength
- Controls weight
- Enhances sleep pattern
- Produces endorphins that lift moods and emotions
- Improves the quality of daily living

Stop thinking that exercises can aggravate stiffness and pains in your joints. Truth is, lack of exercise worsens them. It is vital to strengthen the surrounding tissues and muscles around bones to help joints handle the constant pressures.

So, what kind of physical workout do you need to improve the strength of your bones? The best ones are a combination of aerobic, stretching, and strength exercises.

Endurance exercises or Aerobics

Moderate-intensity aerobic exercises are the most effective and safest for people with arthritis. These types of workouts aid overall fitness by improving cardiovascular health, providing more energy and stamina, and controlling weight.

Low-impact aerobic exercises for joints are walking, swimming, water aerobics, dancing, group exercise classes, gardening, bicycling, and using an elliptical machine.

Aim for 150 minutes of moderate-to-intense aerobic exercises every week. Split them into 10- to 15-minute exercises to prevent joint pressure, especially during the initial stage of the workout.

Strengthening exercises

They support and build strong muscles. They also protect bone joints. Examples are weight training, isometrics, calisthenics, and the use of resistance bands.

Start your exercise regimen with a 3-day-a-week program to improve muscle and bone strength. Remember to avoid exercising the same group of muscles for two consecutive days. Get one day of rest between workouts.

If you feel pain in the joints or they become swollen, rest for a day or two to ensure the condition does not worsen.

Range-of-motion exercises

They relieve stiffness and allow a full range of joint motions. Examples of these movements are forward and backward shoulder rolls and raising both arms over the head. Do them every day.

Other activities that can improve joint condition are:

Body awareness exercises

Yoga, Tai Chi, and other gentle forms of body-mind exercises improve balance and coordination, sustain good body posture, and promote overall relaxation.

One precaution—before practicing any of them make sure to inform the instructor about your arthritic condition to prevent positions or poses that can aggravate it.

Daily activities

Walking the dog, mowing the lawn, raking leaves and other light chores help you exercise the joints.

How much exercise do you need to reap the benefits:

Daily exercising is the best. Short sessions within a week or a day are also good because results are cumulative. Doing 3 ten-minute walks in one day and a 30-minute walk gives similar results.

How intense is the exercise?

Begin slow and easy. Aim for moderate to intense workout.

Take a talk test to measure the level of intensity you can handle. If you need to pause for a breath after saying a few words while exercising, you are having a vigorous-intensity workout. If you can sing while exercising, you are doing a moderate-intensity workout.

Recommended time frames:

- 150-minute exercise weekly of moderate-intensity aerobic exercises or 30-minute exercises 5 times per week.
- 75-minute vigorous-intensity aerobic exercises every week
- combination of moderate-vigorous exercises

Common mistakes to avoid during exercises:

Now that you are committing yourself to be physically active, remember these top fitness mistakes that can do more harm than good to your joints.

Skipping warm-ups

Warm-up raises the body temperature and increases blood flow which loosens up muscles. Without them, you risk potential joint pains and injuries after exercising.

One simple warm-up is a 5-minute march around the room.

No stretching

Stretching sustains the muscles' ability to make a full range of motions. Flexibility plays a major role in preparing the body for aerobic activities especially if you are suffering from joint problems.

The best stretching exercise is the hamstring stretch. It alleviates tightness in the hamstring which is the main cause of misalignment in the knee and pelvis.

Forgetting cool-downs

Proper cool down involves doing long stretches and deep breathing techniques. They restore normal heart rate, blood pressure, and breathing. They also improve the flexibility of joints and muscles.

Doing excessive puffs and huffs

Intense exercises put your body in an anaerobic state. This causes discomfort in joints and muscles. It makes you huff and puff during the workout because your body is not getting enough oxygen.

Using the heaviest dumbbells

Weight training exercises improve stamina and increase energy. However, overdoing them can damage the joint tissues.

In weight training, you will experience fatigue on the 12th or 15th repetition whether you are lifting a 100-pound or 1-pound weight. Start easy then gradually increase the weights to prevent injury.

Going too easy

Sweating out to achieve a 40-70% heart rate target builds more muscles and sustains energy levels.

People with arthritis should exercise within their pain level. Without tolerable pain during a workout, your exercise is too easy for you. Change the intensity to reap the benefits.

Forgetting to drink more

Avoid dehydration during workouts. Your body needs water to keep the blood circulation and temperature normal. Older people and those with joint pains should constantly hydrate themselves.

Drink 6-8 ounces of water before exercising. Drink after every 15-minute workout to replenish the water that you sweat out.

Not eating enough before exercising

Eat 2 hours before the workout to allow proper digestion. Eating near your exercise time makes the body concentrate on digesting the foods instead of keeping the muscles warm and providing the body with oxygen. This can cause nausea and cramps.

Leaning too much

When exercising, avoid resting your arms or leaning on the armrests of stationary equipment because it can aggravate joint pains and affect body posture.

Forgetting to maintain proper body form

Ask your trainer to evaluate your posture or look at yourself in the mirror. People suffering from osteoarthritis or rheumatoid arthritis should maintain proper body positions to prevent injury and pain. Avoid overextending your joints or exercising with improper posture.

Step 5: Seek Complementary Therapies & Home Remedies

There is no single solution that guarantees total relief from arthritic pain. Sometimes, a combination of two or more complementary therapies helps eliminate chronic pains. Other times, simple and natural remedies bring more relief than taking medication.

Complementary Therapy Treatments

- *Acupuncture*: It relieves arthritis pain and inflammation of joints. This ancient method improves the condition of patients who are experiencing moderate to severe pain.
- *Massage*: A Swedish full-body massage that uses slow strokes and pressures to release tension knots on deeper muscle tissues bringing instant relief and relaxation. Another beneficial massage is the myofascial release technique. It uses long, stretching hand strokes to release tension around the connective tissues of muscles.
- *Homeopathy*: It treats chronic osteoarthritis and rheumatoid arthritis by reducing or relieving pains in the ankles, toes, fingers, and hands.

Relaxation Techniques

- *Aromatherapy*: It uses essential oils that provide soothing and anti-inflammatory effects. It eases joint pains.
- *Meditation*: It helps patients handle and manage symptoms of arthritis by keeping the body and mind relaxed.

Psychotherapy Techniques

- *Hypnosis*: This practice helps people suffering from arthritis shift their attention away from pain. Under hypnotic states, they allow their conscious mind to take a break and reach a deep, relaxed state.
- *Biofeedback*: This technique helps patients control their bodies' responses to pain triggers. Learning the technique to control heart rate and breathing empowers them to manage pain and other physical reactions.

Home Remedies

Heat & Cold Methods

Heat eases pain by increasing blood flow. It reduces inflammation and relaxes tight muscles. It eliminates lactic acid and other waste substances that can cause soreness, and stiffness of joints.

Cold helps reduce blood flow which can cause swelling. It inhibits inflammatory chemicals and slows down pain-signal transmission through nerves. It aids in after-exercise swelling and pain or treats injury within 48-72 hours after the incident.

- *Ice Massage*: Rub ice cubes in small circles over affected areas to slow down pain signals, inhibit the production of inflammatory markers, and reduce swelling. Do this for 5-10 minutes several times a day.
- *Warm bath*: Warm water relaxes the muscles and joints. It stimulates blood flow and significantly aids frozen joints and stiff muscles.

7-Day Sample Meal Plan

We've discussed various ways to manage and alleviate symptoms of arthritis, now let's look at a sample meal plan that can help in reducing inflammation and pain. The following is a 7-day sample meal plan for a person suffering from arthritis:

Sunday

Breakfast: Gingerbread Oatmeal

Lunch: Quinoa and Black Bean Salad

Dinner: Lemon Rosemary Chicken with Mediterranean Vegetables

Monday

Breakfast: Turmeric Ginger Oatmeal

Lunch: Broccoli and Almond Soup

Dinner: Sweet Potato and Chickpea Curry

Tuesday

Breakfast: Kale and Avocado Smoothie

Lunch: Salmon with Walnut-Parsley Pesto

Dinner: Poached Eggs with Curry Potatoes

Wednesday

Breakfast: Chia Seed Pudding with Mixed Berries (Soak chia seeds in almond milk overnight, sweeten with a touch of honey, and top with mixed berries before serving)

Lunch: Grilled Vegetable Salad with Olive Oil and Lemon Dressing

Dinner: Salmon with Walnut-Parsley Pesto, Spinach, Apple, and Walnut Salad

Thursday

Breakfast: Berry Antioxidant Smoothie

Lunch: Avocado and Egg Salad on Whole Grain Bread

Dinner: Stuffed Bell Peppers with Quinoa and Vegetables

Friday

Breakfast: Apple Cinnamon Oatmeal

Lunch: Carrot Ginger Soup

Dinner: Baked Cod with a Herb Crust

Saturday

Breakfast: Spinach and Mushroom Omelette

Lunch: Beetroot and Goat Cheese Salad

Dinner: Roasted Chicken Thighs with Garlic and Herbs

Simple Recipes for People with Arthritis

Now that you have a sample meal plan, let's explore some simple recipes that can help manage arthritis symptoms:

Lemon Rosemary Chicken

Ingredients:

- 4 boneless, skinless chicken breasts
- 2 tablespoons olive oil
- 2 lemons, one juiced and one sliced
- 2 cloves garlic, minced
- 2 tablespoons fresh rosemary leaves, chopped (or 1 tablespoon dried rosemary)
- Salt (preferably sea salt or Himalayan pink salt) to taste
- Freshly ground black pepper to taste

Instructions:

1. Preheat Oven: Preheat your oven to 375°F (190°C).
2. Marinate Chicken: In a bowl, combine the olive oil, lemon juice, minced garlic, rosemary, salt, and pepper. Add the chicken breasts to the marinade, ensuring they are well coated. Let them marinate for at least 30 minutes in the refrigerator. If you have time, marinating for a couple of hours can enhance the flavors even more.
3. Prepare Baking Dish: Lightly grease a baking dish with a bit of olive oil. Arrange the lemon slices in a single layer at the bottom of the dish.
4. Arrange Chicken: Remove the chicken from the marinade (reserve the marinade) and place them on top

of the lemon slices in the baking dish. Pour the remaining marinade over the chicken.
5. Bake: Place the baking dish in the preheated oven and bake for 25-30 minutes, or until the chicken is thoroughly cooked and no longer pink in the middle. The internal temperature should reach 165°F (74°C) when checked with a meat thermometer.
6. Rest and Serve: Once done, let the chicken rest for a few minutes before serving. This allows the juices to be redistributed, making the chicken more tender. Serve hot, garnished with additional fresh rosemary and lemon slices if desired.
7. Serving Suggestion: Pair this Lemon Rosemary Chicken with a side of steamed or roasted vegetables, such as broccoli, Brussels sprouts, or a mixed green salad, to round out an anti-inflammatory meal.

Mediterranean Vegetables

Ingredients:

- 1 cup baby carrots
- 1 cup snow peas, trimmed
- 1 cup baby corn, halved lengthwise
- 1 cup cherry tomatoes, halved
- 2 tablespoons extra virgin olive oil
- 2 teaspoons turmeric
- 1 tablespoon balsamic vinegar
- 3 garlic cloves, minced
- A couple of sprigs of fresh thyme (or 1 teaspoon dried thyme)
- Salt (preferably sea salt or Himalayan pink salt) to taste
- Freshly ground black pepper to taste

Instructions:

1. Preheat Oven: Preheat your oven to 400°F (200°C).
2. Prepare Vegetables: Mix together the baby carrots, snow peas, baby corn, and cherry tomatoes in a sizeable mixing bowl.
3. Season: In a small bowl, whisk together the extra virgin olive oil, turmeric, balsamic vinegar, and minced garlic until well combined. Pour this mixture over the vegetables in the mixing bowl. Add the thyme, salt, and pepper, then toss everything together

until the vegetables are evenly coated with the seasoning.
4. Roast: Spread the seasoned vegetables out in a single layer on a baking sheet lined with parchment paper. Ensure they are not overcrowded to allow them to roast evenly.
5. Bake: Place the baking sheet in the preheated oven and roast the vegetables for about 20-25 minutes, or until tender and lightly caramelized around the edges. Halfway through the roasting time, give the vegetables a gentle stir to ensure even cooking.
6. Serve: Once the vegetables are roasted to perfection, remove them from the oven and let them cool for a few minutes. Taste and adjust seasoning if necessary. Serve warm as a side dish or incorporate them into other meals as desired.
7. Serving Suggestion: These roasted vegetables are delicious as a side dish for any protein, such as chicken, fish, or tofu. They can also be added to salads, pasta dishes, or grain bowls for a nutritious and flavorful boost.

Poached Eggs with Curry Potatoes

Ingredients:

- 1 lb (about 450g) small potatoes, scrubbed and halved
- 2 tablespoons extra virgin olive oil
- 1 teaspoon turmeric
- 1 teaspoon cumin
- 1/2 teaspoon coriander
- Salt (preferably sea salt or Himalayan pink salt) to taste
- Freshly ground black pepper to taste
- 4 large eggs
- 2 teaspoons white vinegar (for poaching eggs)
- Fresh cilantro (coriander leaves), chopped for garnish
- Optional: chili flakes for extra heat

Instructions:

1. Preheat Oven: Preheat your oven to 400°F (200°C).
2. Season Potatoes: In a large mixing bowl, combine the halved potatoes, extra virgin olive oil, turmeric, cumin, coriander, salt, and black pepper. Toss until the potatoes are evenly coated with the oil and spices.
3. Roast Potatoes: Spread the seasoned potatoes on a baking sheet lined with parchment paper in a single layer. Roast in the preheated oven for about 25-30 minutes or until they are tender and golden brown.

Halfway through, flip the potatoes to ensure even roasting.
4. Poach Eggs: While the potatoes are roasting, bring a medium-sized pot of water to a gentle simmer. Add the white vinegar. Crack each egg into a small cup or bowl and gently slide them into the simmering water one at a time. Poach the eggs for about 3-4 minutes for soft yolks or longer for firmer yolks. Remove the eggs with a slotted spoon and place them on a paper towel to drain.
5. Serve: Divide the roasted curry potatoes among plates. Top each serving with a poached egg. Garnish with chopped fresh cilantro and, if desired, a sprinkle of chili flakes for added heat.
6. Enjoy: Serve immediately, enjoying the blend of flavors and textures.
7. Serving Suggestion: This dish would pair well with a side of toasted naan bread and a refreshing cucumber raita dip. For added protein, you could also serve it with grilled chicken or tofu on the side.

Gingerbread Oatmeal

Ingredients:

- 1 cup steel-cut oats (gluten-free if necessary)
- 4 cups water
- 1 cup non-dairy milk (such as oat milk or almond milk)
- 1/2 teaspoon ground cinnamon
- 1/4 teaspoon ground cloves
- 1/4 teaspoon ground ginger
- 1/4 teaspoon ground nutmeg
- 1 tablespoon molasses (for authentic gingerbread flavor and added sweetness)
- Optional toppings: chopped nuts (like walnuts or almonds), fresh berries, a dollop of unsweetened applesauce, or a sprinkle of chia seeds

Instructions:

1. Cook Oats: In a large saucepan, bring 4 cups of water to a boil. Add the steel-cut oats and stir. Reduce the heat to a simmer and cook uncovered for about 20-30 minutes, stirring occasionally until the oats are tender and have absorbed most of the water.
2. Add Spices and Molasses: Once the oats are nearly done, stir in the non-dairy milk, cinnamon, cloves, ginger, nutmeg, and molasses. Continue to cook for another 5-10 minutes, stirring frequently, until the

mixture is creamy and all the flavors are well combined.
3. Adjust Consistency: If the oatmeal is too thick for your liking, you can add a little more non-dairy milk until you reach your desired consistency.
4. Serve: Divide the oatmeal into bowls. Garnish with your choice of optional toppings for additional texture and flavor.
5. Enjoy: Serve warm for a cozy and nutritious breakfast.
6. Serving Suggestion: For added protein, serve this gingerbread oatmeal with a side of grilled chicken or tofu. Alternatively, you can also top it with a spoonful of your favorite nut butter for a delicious and filling breakfast option.

Turmeric Ginger Oatmeal

Ingredients:

- 1 cup rolled oats (use gluten-free oats if necessary)
- 2 cups almond milk or any plant-based milk of your choice
- 1 tsp turmeric powder
- ½ tsp ginger powder or 1 tsp fresh grated ginger
- ½ tsp cinnamon powder
- A pinch of black pepper (to enhance the absorption of turmeric)
- 1 tbsp maple syrup or honey (optional, for sweetness)
- Fresh berries (such as blueberries and strawberries) for topping
- A handful of chopped nuts (walnuts, almonds) for added texture and nutrients
- Optional: 1 tsp chia seeds for extra fiber

Instructions:

1. Combine Ingredients: In a medium saucepan, combine the rolled oats and almond milk. Stir in the turmeric, ginger, cinnamon, and a pinch of black pepper. If you're using fresh grated ginger, make sure it is finely minced or grated so it integrates well into the oatmeal.
2. Cook Oatmeal: Place the saucepan over medium heat. Bring the mixture to a gentle boil, then reduce the heat to low. Simmer for 5-7 minutes, stirring occasionally,

until the oats are fully cooked and have absorbed most of the liquid. If you prefer a thinner consistency, feel free to add a little more almond milk as it cooks.
3. Sweeten and Serve: Once the oatmeal is cooked to your liking, remove it from the heat. Stir in the maple syrup or honey if using. This step is optional and can be adjusted based on your preferred level of sweetness.
4. Add Toppings: Pour the oatmeal into bowls. Top with fresh berries, chopped nuts, and chia seeds if desired. These toppings not only add flavor and texture but also pack in additional nutrients beneficial for an arthritis-friendly diet.
5. Enjoy: Serve warm and enjoy a nourishing start to your day.
6. Serving Suggestion: For extra protein, add protein powder or nut butter. Perfect for meal prep - make a bigger batch and store leftovers in the fridge for quick breakfasts all week. Use as a base for overnight oats: mix ingredients in a jar, refrigerate overnight, and top with favorite toppings in the morning for an easy breakfast on the go.

Kale and Avocado Smoothie

Ingredients:

- 2 cups fresh kale leaves, stems removed
- 1 ripe avocado, pitted and scooped
- 1/2 cup parsley leaves
- 1 banana, preferably frozen for a creamy texture
- 1/2 cup blueberries (fresh or frozen)
- 1 tablespoon chia seeds
- 1 cup dairy-free milk (almond, coconut, or oat milk work well)
- 1/2 medium apple, cored and chopped (for added sweetness and fiber)
- Optional: 1 tablespoon fresh ginger, grated (for extra anti-inflammatory benefits)
- Ice cubes (optional, for a colder smoothie)

Instructions:

1. Prepare the Ingredients: Wash the kale and parsley leaves thoroughly. Chop the kale into smaller pieces if necessary to make blending easier. Cut the avocado in half, remove the pit, and scoop out the flesh.
2. Blend Greens and Liquid: In a high-powered blender, combine the kale leaves, parsley, and dairy-free milk. Blend on high speed until the greens are fully broken down and you have a smooth mixture.

3. Add Remaining Ingredients: To the blender, add the avocado, banana, blueberries, chia seeds, chopped apple, and grated ginger (if using). If you prefer a colder smoothie, you can also add some ice cubes at this stage.
4. Blend Until Smooth: Blend everything together on high speed until the smoothie reaches a creamy and smooth consistency. If the smoothie is too thick, you can add a little more dairy-free milk to reach your desired consistency.
5. Taste and Adjust: Give your smoothie a taste and adjust as needed. If you prefer it sweeter, you could add a little more banana or a splash of maple syrup. If it's too thick, add more dairy-free milk.
6. Serve Immediately: Pour the smoothie into glasses and enjoy immediately. The quicker you consume it after blending, the more nutrients you'll benefit from.
7. Serving Suggestion: This smoothie is a great way to start your day with a boost of nutrients and energy. It pairs well with a protein-packed breakfast such as avocado toast or scrambled eggs. You can also enjoy it as a mid-day snack or post-workout refuel.

Quinoa and Black Bean Salad

Ingredients:

- 1 cup quinoa (dry)
- 2 cups water or vegetable broth (for cooking quinoa)
- 1 can (15 ounces) black beans, drained and rinsed
- 1 cup corn kernels (fresh, frozen and thawed, or canned)
- 1 medium red bell pepper, diced
- 1/2 cup red onion, finely chopped
- 1/2 cup fresh cilantro, chopped
- 1 avocado, diced
- 1/4 cup olive oil
- Juice of 2 limes (about 3 tablespoons)
- 1/2 teaspoon ground cumin
- 1/2 teaspoon ground coriander
- Salt and pepper to taste
- Optional: 1 teaspoon chili powder for a little kick

Instructions:

1. Cook the Quinoa: Rinse the quinoa under cold water in a fine-mesh strainer. In a medium saucepan, bring 2 cups of water or vegetable broth to a boil. Add the quinoa, reduce heat to low, cover, and simmer for about 15 minutes, or until all the liquid is absorbed. Remove from heat and let it sit covered for 5 minutes. Fluff with a fork and allow it to cool.

2. Prepare the Salad Ingredients: While the quinoa is cooling, prepare the rest of your salad ingredients. Drain and rinse the black beans, chop the red bell pepper, red onion, and cilantro, and dice the avocado. If using frozen corn, ensure it's thawed.
3. Make the Dressing: In a small bowl, whisk together the olive oil, lime juice, ground cumin, ground coriander, salt, pepper, and optional chili powder. Adjust the seasoning according to your taste.
4. Combine the Salad: Mix together the cooled quinoa, black beans, corn, red bell pepper, red onion, and cilantro in a sizable bowl. Pour the dressing over the salad and gently toss to combine everything evenly.
5. Add Avocado: Gently fold in the diced avocado last to prevent it from getting mushy.
6. Chill and Serve: Let the salad chill in the refrigerator for at least 30 minutes before serving. This allows the flavors to meld together. Give it a quick toss before serving.
7. Serving Suggestion: Serve the quinoa salad as a side dish, or add some protein like grilled chicken or shrimp to make it a complete meal. You can also serve it on top of some leafy greens for added nutrition and texture.

Salmon with Walnut-Parsley Pesto

Ingredients:

- 4 salmon fillets (about 6 ounces each)
- 1 cup fresh parsley leaves, tightly packed
- 1/2 cup walnuts, toasted
- 2 cloves garlic, minced
- 1/4 cup extra-virgin olive oil, plus extra for drizzling
- Juice and zest of 1 lemon
- Salt and freshly ground black pepper, to taste

Instructions:

1. Preheat the Oven: Start by preheating your oven to 400°F (200°C). Line a baking tray with parchment paper for easy cleanup.
2. Make the Walnut-Parsley Pesto: In a food processor, combine the parsley leaves, toasted walnuts, minced garlic, lemon juice, and zest. Pulse until the ingredients are finely chopped. While the processor is running, slowly pour in the 1/4 cup of olive oil. Continue processing until the mixture becomes a coarse paste. Season with salt and pepper to taste. If the pesto is too thick, you can add a little more olive oil to reach your desired consistency.
3. Prepare the Salmon: Place the salmon fillets on the prepared baking tray. Drizzle a little olive oil over each fillet and season with salt and pepper. Use a spoon to

spread a generous layer of walnut-parsley pesto over each fillet.
4. Bake the Salmon: Place the baking tray in the preheated oven and bake for about 12-15 minutes, or until the salmon is cooked through and flakes easily with a fork. The cooking time may vary depending on the thickness of the fillets.
5. Serve: Once the salmon is cooked, remove it from the oven. You can serve the salmon fillets with a side of steamed vegetables or a fresh salad for a complete meal.
6. Serving Suggestion: This walnut-parsley pesto is a versatile topping that can be used for other proteins like chicken or shrimp. You can also mix it with your favorite pasta for a delicious and easy weeknight dinner. Store any leftover pesto in an airtight container in the fridge for up to 3 days.

Sweet Potato and Chickpea Curry

Ingredients:

- 2 medium sweet potatoes, peeled and cubed
- 1 can (about 15 oz) chickpeas, drained and rinsed
- 1 large onion, finely chopped
- 2 cloves garlic, minced
- 1-inch piece of ginger, grated
- 1 can (about 14 oz) coconut milk
- 2 tablespoons tomato paste
- 1 tablespoon curry powder
- 1 teaspoon turmeric powder
- 1 teaspoon cumin powder
- 1/2 teaspoon chili powder (adjust to taste)
- 2 tablespoons coconut oil
- Salt to taste
- Fresh cilantro, chopped, for garnish
- Cooked brown rice or quinoa, for serving

Instructions:

1. Prepare the ingredients: Heat the coconut oil in a large pan over medium heat. Add the onion, garlic, and ginger, sautéing until the onions become translucent and fragrant, about 5 minutes.
2. Spice it up: Stir in the curry powder, turmeric, cumin, and chili powder. Cook for another minute until the spices are well combined and aromatic.

3. Combine: Add the sweet potatoes to the pan, stirring well to coat them with the spices. Cook for about 2-3 minutes.
4. Simmer: Pour in the coconut milk and add the tomato paste. Bring the mixture to a simmer, then reduce the heat to low. Cover and let it cook for about 10 minutes.
5. Add chickpeas: Stir in the chickpeas and continue to simmer, covered, for another 10-15 minutes, or until the sweet potatoes are tender and the curry has thickened. Adjust salt to taste.
6. Serve: Serve the curry warm over cooked brown rice or quinoa, garnished with fresh cilantro.
7. Serving Suggestion: This sweet potato and chickpea curry is tasty solo, or pair it with naan bread or pita for a heartier meal. Add roasted veggies or tofu for extra texture and flavor. Ideal for leftovers, make a big batch to enjoy all week. Save some for tomorrow's lunch! Get creative and have fun with this versatile dish.

Salmon with Walnut-Parsley Pesto, Spinach, Apple, and Walnut Salad

Ingredients

For the Salmon:

- 4 salmon fillets (about 6 ounces each)
- 1 tablespoon olive oil
- Salt and pepper, to taste

For the Walnut-Parsley Pesto:

- 1 cup fresh parsley leaves
- 1/2 cup walnuts, plus more for garnish
- 2 garlic cloves, minced
- 1/4 cup grated Parmesan cheese
- 1/2 cup extra-virgin olive oil
- Salt and pepper, to taste

For the Spinach, Apple, and Walnut Salad:

- 4 cups baby spinach
- 1 apple, thinly sliced
- 1/4 cup walnuts, roughly chopped
- 2 tablespoons balsamic vinegar
- 1 tablespoon honey
- 3 tablespoons extra-virgin olive oil
- Salt and pepper, to taste

Instructions:

Salmon:

1. Preheat the oven to 400°F (200°C).
2. Season the salmon fillets with salt and pepper, then brush them with olive oil.
3. Place the salmon on a baking sheet lined with parchment paper, and bake for 12-15 minutes, or until the salmon flakes easily with a fork.
4. Remove from the oven and let it rest.

Walnut-Parsley Pesto:

1. Place the parsley, walnuts, garlic, and Parmesan cheese into a food processor and pulse until they reach a coarsely chopped texture.
2. While the processor is in operation, gradually incorporate the olive oil until the mixture achieves a smooth consistency. Add salt and pepper according to your preference.

Spinach, Apple, and Walnut Salad:

1. Mix the baby spinach, sliced apple, and chopped walnuts together in a big bowl.
2. In a small bowl, whisk together the balsamic vinegar, honey, and olive oil. Season with salt and pepper to taste.

3. Drizzle the dressing over the salad and toss to combine.

Assembly:

1. Place a generous serving of the Spinach, Apple, and Walnut Salad on each plate.
2. Top with a salmon fillet and a spoonful of the Walnut-Parsley Pesto.
3. Garnish with additional walnuts if desired.
4. Serving Suggestion: This Spinach, Apple, and Walnut Salad with Baked Salmon is a light and healthy meal for lunch or dinner. Enjoy it alone or with a side dish. Perfect for summer or a picnic. Try it to impress friends and family! For a quick meal, make this salad next time.

Broccoli and Almond Soup

Ingredients:

- 2 cups fresh broccoli florets
- 1/2 cup raw almonds, plus more for garnish (optional)
- 1 medium onion, finely chopped
- 2 cloves garlic, minced
- 2 tablespoons extra virgin olive oil
- 4 cups vegetable broth
- 1 cup almond milk (unsweetened)
- 1/2 teaspoon turmeric powder
- 1/2 teaspoon ground cumin
- Salt and pepper, to taste
- A handful of fresh spinach leaves (optional for extra nutrition)

Instructions:

1. Prep the Broccoli and Almonds: In a large pot, heat 1 tablespoon of olive oil over medium heat. Add the broccoli florets and cook for about 5 minutes, or until they start to soften. Remove from the pot and set aside. In the same pot, add the almonds and toast them lightly for about 3 minutes, then remove and set aside.
2. Sauté the Aromatics: In the same pot, add the remaining tablespoon of olive oil along with the chopped onion and minced garlic. Sauté until the onion

becomes translucent and the garlic is fragrant about 2-3 minutes.

3. Simmer the Soup: Return the broccoli to the pot and add the vegetable broth, almond milk, turmeric, and cumin. Bring the mixture to a boil, then reduce the heat and let it simmer for about 15-20 minutes, or until the broccoli is completely tender.
4. Blend the Soup: Carefully transfer the soup mixture to a blender, adding most of the toasted almonds (reserve some for garnish if desired). Blend until the soup reaches a smooth and creamy consistency. If the soup is too thick, you can add a little more vegetable broth or almond milk to reach your preferred consistency.
5. Season and Serve: Return the blended soup to the pot and reheat if necessary. Taste and adjust the seasoning with salt and pepper. If using, stir in a handful of fresh spinach leaves until wilted.
6. Garnish and Enjoy: Serve the soup hot, garnished with the reserved toasted almonds. This adds a delightful crunch and nutty flavor to each bite.

7. Serving Suggestion: Pair this delicious broccoli and almond soup with crusty bread or a light salad for a satisfying, healthy meal. Add cooked rice or quinoa for extra filling. Serve the soup as a starter at dinner parties in small cups or shot glasses for an elegant touch. Get creative with garnishes like fresh herbs, croutons, or a drizzle of olive oil for added flavor and texture. Make this soup your own!

Conclusion

Congratulations on reaching the conclusion of our comprehensive guide on arthritis and the pivotal role that diet plays in managing this condition. By now, you've armed yourself with valuable insights into how certain foods can alleviate arthritis symptoms, reduce inflammation, and potentially slow down the disease's progression. Your commitment to understanding and applying these principles is a testament to your dedication to improving your health and quality of life.

Arthritis, as you've learned, is not a singular disease but a complex family of musculoskeletal disorders that affect millions worldwide. Its manifestations can be diverse, ranging from mild discomfort to debilitating pain, significantly impacting daily activities and overall well-being. However, the empowering takeaway from our guide is that you have the power to influence the course of your arthritis through dietary choices. This realization marks a critical step in reclaiming control over your health.

The anti-inflammatory diet, rich in fruits, vegetables, whole grains, lean protein, and healthy fats, isn't just a blueprint for managing arthritis; it's a formula for overall wellness. Incorporating these nutrient-dense foods into your daily routine can lead to noticeable improvements in your symptoms and, importantly, enhance your energy levels, mood, and cognitive function. The Mediterranean diet, in particular, has been highlighted for its beneficial effects on reducing inflammation and supporting joint health.

Moreover, understanding the foods to avoid is equally crucial. Processed foods, sugars, and certain fats can exacerbate inflammation and counteract the positive strides you're making with healthier choices. Being mindful of these triggers and learning to navigate social situations and cravings is a skill that will serve you well on this journey.

Hydration and moderation are key themes that we've emphasized throughout this guide. Drinking plenty of water and moderating the consumption of alcohol and caffeine can further support your body's natural defenses against inflammation and pain. Remember, small, consistent changes are more sustainable and effective than drastic overhauls that are hard to maintain.

As you move forward, equipped with this knowledge, remember that patience and persistence are your allies. The benefits of a diet tailored to managing arthritis might not be immediate, but with time, you will likely notice a positive shift in how you feel. Listen to your body, and don't hesitate to consult with healthcare professionals to tailor these guidelines to your specific needs and circumstances.

In closing, we commend you for taking this significant step toward a healthier, more vibrant life despite the challenges of arthritis. Your proactive approach to learning and implementing an arthritis-friendly diet is inspiring. It's a powerful reminder that, although we may not have control over every aspect of our health, there are meaningful actions we can take to improve our well-being.

Remember, this guide is not the end but a beginning—a launching pad for a lifelong journey of discovery, resilience, and self-care. Continue to explore, adjust, and refine your dietary choices. Share your experiences with others, and let your journey be a beacon of hope and encouragement for those navigating similar paths.

FAQ

What foods are recommended for managing arthritis pain?

Foods rich in anti-inflammatory properties and omega-3s are recommended for arthritis pain. Include fatty fish (salmon, mackerel, sardines), cherries, leafy greens, garlic, olive oil, nuts, and beans. Add whole grains, fruits, and veggies to reduce inflammation and support joint health.

Are there any foods I should avoid if I have arthritis?

Certain foods can worsen inflammation and should be limited or avoided, like processed foods, saturated fats, refined sugars, dairy products, red meat, and alcohol, which can increase inflammation and pain in some individuals.

Can changing my diet really help with arthritis symptoms?

Indeed, though diet alone may not cure arthritis, adding anti-inflammatory foods can greatly reduce inflammation, ease pain, and enhance joint function. A well-rounded, healthy diet can also boost overall health and potentially delay disease progression.

Is there a specific diet plan I should follow for my type of arthritis?

While there's no universal diet for arthritis, the Mediterranean diet is often suggested for its anti-inflammatory foods. Tailor your diet to your needs and arthritis type. For example, those with gout may need to limit purine-rich foods such as red meat and seafood.

How can I start an arthritis-friendly diet?

Start by adding anti-inflammatory foods like fatty fish, fruits, veggies, nuts, and whole grains to your diet. Cut back on processed foods, sugars, and saturated fats. Keep a food diary to monitor how foods impact your symptoms.

Can supplements and vitamins help with arthritis?

Certain supplements like omega-3s, vitamin D, and glucosamine may ease arthritis symptoms for some. Consult a healthcare pro before beginning any regimen, as supplements can interact with meds or not be suitable for all.

Are there any other lifestyle changes that can help with arthritis besides diet?

Diet changes, a healthy weight, being active, and regular exercise can help arthritis symptoms. Low-impact activities like walking, swimming, or yoga improve joint flexibility and strength without worsening pain. Manage stress and get enough sleep to impact inflammation and well-being.

References and Helpful Links

Arthritis. (n.d.). Johns Hopkins Medicine. https://www.hopkinsmedicine.org/health/conditions-and-diseases/arthritis#:~:text=Arthritis%20means%20redness%20and%20swelling,tendons%2C%20ligaments%2C%20or%20bones.

Barrell, A. (2024, January 25). What is the best diet for osteoarthritis? https://www.medicalnewstoday.com/articles/322603

Arthritis cost Statistics | CDC. (n.d.). https://www.cdc.gov/arthritis/data_statistics/cost.htm

Arthritis - Symptoms and causes - Mayo Clinic. (2023, August 29). Mayo Clinic. https://www.mayoclinic.org/diseases-conditions/arthritis/symptoms-causes/syc-20350772

The Ultimate Arthritis Diet | Arthritis Foundation. (n.d.). https://www.arthritis.org/health-wellness/healthy-living/nutrition/anti-inflammatory/the-ultimate-arthritis-diet

5 ways to manage arthritis | CDC. (n.d.). https://www.cdc.gov/arthritis/basics/management.htm

Rd, E. L. M. (2024, January 14). Rheumatoid arthritis meal plan. EatingWell.

https://www.eatingwell.com/article/7866119/rheumatoid-arthritis-diet-plan/

Ld, S. S. M. R. (2022, April 13). 7-Day meal plan to Fight inflammation: Recipes and more. Healthline. https://www.healthline.com/health/rheumatoid-arthritis/seven-day-meal-plan

www.ingramcontent.com/pod-product-compliance
Lightning Source LLC
LaVergne TN
LVHW012034060526
838201LV00061B/4601